Metabolic Health Guide Made Easy for Beginners

Managing Stress for Better Metabolic Health

By

Dane Elio

Table of Contents

CHAPTER 1

Introduction to Metabolic Health

1.1 What is Metabolic Health

Metabolic health refers to the state of balance and efficiency within the body's metabolic processes. It encompasses a range of physiological functions that include the conversion of food into energy, the utilization of nutrients for various bodily functions, and the regulation of factors like blood sugar, cholesterol levels, and more. Metabolic health isn't solely about having a fast metabolism; it's about having a well-functioning metabolism that supports overall well-being.

At its core, metabolic health involves the harmonious interaction of several systems, including the digestive, endocrine, and cardiovascular systems. When these systems function optimally, the body can effectively extract energy from the food we eat and distribute it to cells for various functions, such as growth, repair, and maintaining bodily processes.

1.2 Why is Metabolic Health Important

Metabolic health is of paramount importance as it directly influences various aspects of our well-being. A well-functioning metabolism is crucial for maintaining a healthy body weight, as it determines how efficiently our body burns calories. When metabolic processes are disrupted, it can lead to weight gain, obesity, and related health issues such as diabetes, cardiovascular disease, and more.

Metabolic health plays a significant role in regulating blood sugar levels. Balanced blood sugar levels are essential to prevent insulin resistance and type 2 diabetes. Insulin, a hormone produced by the pancreas, is responsible for facilitating the uptake of glucose into cells for energy. Poor metabolic health can lead to insulin resistance, where cells become less responsive to insulin, resulting in elevated blood sugar levels and potential long-term health complications.

Beyond weight management and blood sugar regulation, metabolic health affects lipid metabolism. The balance of cholesterol and triglycerides in the bloodstream is crucial for cardiovascular health. Imbalances can contribute to atherosclerosis (hardening of the arteries) and an increased risk of heart disease.

1.3 How Does Metabolism Work

Metabolism is the intricate network of chemical reactions that occur within cells to sustain life. It involves two main processes: anabolism and catabolism. Anabolism encompasses the building of molecules and structures needed for cell growth, repair, and function. Catabolism involves the breakdown of complex molecules into simpler compounds, releasing energy in the process.

The primary unit of energy currency in metabolism is adenosine triphosphate (ATP). When food is consumed, it's broken down into macronutrients: carbohydrates, proteins, and fats. Carbohydrates are converted into glucose, proteins into amino acids, and fats into fatty acids and glycerol. These components enter various metabolic pathways to produce ATP and other molecules that cells require.

The basal metabolic rate (BMR) represents the energy expended by the body at rest to maintain basic functions like breathing, circulating blood, and cellular activity. Physical activity, thermogenesis (heat production), and digestion also contribute to the overall energy expenditure.

Metabolism is tightly regulated by hormones, including insulin, glucagon, thyroid hormones, and more. These hormones influence how cells use and store nutrients, ensuring that energy is available when needed and stored appropriately for times of scarcity.

understanding metabolic health is pivotal for maintaining overall well-being. A balanced and efficient metabolism supports weight management, blood sugar regulation, and cardiovascular health. By comprehending the fundamental principles of metabolism and adopting healthy lifestyle habits, individuals can work towards achieving and sustaining optimal metabolic health.

CHAPTER 2

Understanding the Basics of Metabolism

2.1 An Overview of Energy Metabolism

Energy metabolism is the intricate process through which the body converts the energy stored in the foods we consume into a usable form, primarily adenosine triphosphate (ATP). ATP serves as the energy currency of the body, powering various cellular activities and processes necessary for life.

The energy obtained from our diet comes from macronutrients: carbohydrates, proteins, and fats.

Carbohydrates are the body's preferred source of quick energy, and they are broken down into glucose during digestion. Glucose can be used immediately for energy or stored as glycogen in the liver and muscles for later use. When glycogen stores are full, excess glucose is converted into fat for long-term storage.

Proteins, composed of amino acids, serve as building blocks for various tissues in the body. If there is an excess of protein intake beyond what the body needs for repair and growth, the excess amino acids can be converted into glucose or fatty acids, contributing to energy storage.

Fats, in the form of triglycerides, are a dense and efficient storage form of energy. During metabolism, fats are broken down into fatty acids and glycerol. Fatty acids can be used for energy immediately or stored in adipose tissue for later use. They are also integral to many physiological processes, including the formation of cell membranes and the synthesis of hormones.

The process of energy metabolism involves a series of interconnected reactions that take place in various cellular compartments, with enzymes playing a critical role in catalyzing these reactions. These reactions occur in different stages, including glycolysis, the citric acid cycle (Krebs cycle), and oxidative phosphorylation (electron transport chain), which take place in the mitochondria. These stages collectively result in the production of ATP.

2.2 Metabolic Pathways: Breaking Down Nutrients

Metabolic pathways are a series of chemical reactions that convert nutrients from the food we eat into usable energy and other essential molecules. These pathways are highly organized and regulated to ensure efficient energy production and the synthesis of necessary molecules.

1. **Glycolysis**: This pathway takes place in the cytoplasm and involves the breakdown of glucose into pyruvate. It yields a small amount of ATP and NADH, which can be used later in energy production.

2. **Citric Acid Cycle (Krebs Cycle)**: Taking place in the mitochondria, the citric acid cycle further breaks

down pyruvate into carbon dioxide and generates additional ATP, NADH, and FADH2.

3. **Oxidative Phosphorylation (Electron Transport Chain)**: This crucial step occurs in the inner mitochondrial membrane. NADH and FADH2 generated in previous steps donate electrons to the electron transport chain, creating a flow of protons across the mitochondrial membrane. This proton gradient drives the production of ATP through a process called chemiosmosis.

4. **Beta-Oxidation**: In the breakdown of fatty acids, beta-oxidation occurs in the mitochondria. Fatty acids are broken down into acetyl-CoA, which enters the citric acid cycle.

5. **Amino Acid Metabolism**: Amino acids can be converted into intermediates of glycolysis or the citric acid cycle, depending on the specific amino acid and the body's needs. Some amino acids can also be used for gluconeogenesis, the synthesis of glucose.

These pathways don't operate in isolation; they are interconnected and adapt based on the body's energy needs and nutrient availability. The intricate coordination of these pathways ensures that energy production is efficient and responsive to various physiological demands.

understanding energy metabolism and metabolic pathways provides insights into how the body converts nutrients into usable energy and other essential molecules. This knowledge underscores the importance of maintaining a balanced diet to ensure optimal energy production and overall health.

2.3 Role of Hormones in Metabolism

Hormones play a crucial role in regulating various aspects of metabolism. These chemical messengers are produced by glands in the endocrine system and circulate throughout the body, orchestrating the activities of different organs and tissues. Hormones help maintain metabolic homeostasis by influencing processes such as energy utilization, storage, and distribution.

Here are some key hormones and their roles in metabolism:

1. **Insulin**: Produced by the pancreas, insulin is a central hormone in

regulating blood sugar levels. When blood glucose rises after eating, insulin is released to facilitate the uptake of glucose into cells, particularly muscle and adipose tissue. It promotes the conversion of glucose into glycogen for storage in the liver and muscles. Insulin also inhibits the breakdown of stored fat and promotes fat storage, making it a crucial regulator of energy storage.

2. **Glucagon**: Also produced by the pancreas, glucagon has an opposing role to insulin. It is released when blood glucose levels drop, such as between meals or during exercise. Glucagon stimulates the liver to break down glycogen into glucose and release it into the bloodstream. This process, known as glycogenolysis,

helps raise blood sugar levels to provide energy for the body's needs.

3. **Leptin**: Produced by adipose tissue (fat cells), leptin serves as a satiety hormone that communicates the body's energy status to the brain. Higher levels of leptin indicate sufficient energy stores, signaling to the brain to reduce appetite and increase energy expenditure. In cases of obesity, individuals may become resistant to leptin's effects, leading to a disruption in appetite regulation.

4. **Ghrelin**: Ghrelin is produced primarily in the stomach and plays a role in stimulating appetite. It is often referred to as the "hunger hormone" because its levels rise before meals and decrease after

eating. Ghrelin signals to the brain that it's time to eat and contributes to the regulation of meal timing and frequency.

5. **Thyroid Hormones (T3 and T4)**: Produced by the thyroid gland, thyroid hormones play a central role in regulating the basal metabolic rate. They influence the rate at which cells use energy and are involved in many physiological processes, including growth, development, and thermoregulation.

6. **Cortisol**: Produced by the adrenal glands, cortisol is often referred to as the "stress hormone." It plays a role in metabolism by influencing glucose metabolism, promoting gluconeogenesis (glucose synthesis) in the liver, and mobilizing amino acids from

muscle tissue. Chronically elevated cortisol levels, often associated with chronic stress, can lead to metabolic imbalances.

7. **Adiponectin**: Secreted by adipose tissue, adiponectin helps regulate insulin sensitivity and plays a role in lipid metabolism. Higher levels of adiponectin are generally associated with improved insulin sensitivity and a decreased risk of metabolic diseases like type 2 diabetes.

8. **Epinephrine and Norepinephrine**: These hormones are produced by the adrenal glands and are often referred to as the "fight or flight" hormones. They increase heart rate, mobilize energy stores, and promote the breakdown of glycogen for

immediate energy during stressful situations or physical activity.

The interaction of these hormones forms a complex network that helps the body respond to changing energy needs, maintain blood sugar levels, regulate appetite, and store and utilize energy efficiently. Dysregulation of hormonal balance can lead to metabolic disorders, underscoring the importance of maintaining a healthy lifestyle and seeking medical guidance when necessary.

CHAPTER 3

Key Factors Affecting Metabolic Health

3.1 Diet and Nutrition

3.1.1 Macronutrients and Micronutrients

Diet plays a pivotal role in shaping metabolic health. The nutrients we consume can impact energy production, hormonal regulation, and overall metabolic function. Macronutrients, including carbohydrates, proteins, and fats, provide the body with energy and essential building blocks. Micronutrients, such as vitamins and minerals, are required in smaller amounts but are equally critical for various metabolic processes.

Carbohydrates are the body's primary source of energy, providing glucose that fuels cells. Complex carbohydrates from whole grains, fruits, and vegetables offer sustained energy due to their fiber content, while refined carbohydrates from sugary snacks and processed foods can lead to rapid blood sugar spikes and crashes.

Proteins are essential for tissue repair, enzyme production, and maintaining muscle mass. Amino acids, the building blocks of proteins, play a role in metabolism as they can be used for energy when carbohydrate stores are depleted.

Fats are vital for energy storage, hormone production, and cell membrane structure. Unsaturated fats, found in foods like nuts, seeds, and avocados, are healthier choices compared to saturated and trans fats found in fried and processed foods.

Micronutrients, such as vitamins (e.g., vitamin D, B vitamins) and minerals (e.g., calcium, magnesium), support enzymatic reactions, energy production, and overall health. Deficiencies in these micronutrients can disrupt metabolic pathways and lead to health issues.

3.1.2 The Impact of Sugar and Processed Foods

Excessive consumption of added sugars and processed foods has a profound negative impact on metabolic health. High sugar intake can lead to insulin resistance, weight gain, and an increased risk of type 2 diabetes. Processed foods often contain unhealthy fats, excessive sodium, and additives that can contribute to inflammation and metabolic dysfunction.

3.1.3 Importance of Balanced Eating

Balanced eating involves consuming a variety of nutrient-dense foods in appropriate portions. This approach helps maintain steady blood sugar levels, prevents overeating, and provides essential nutrients for optimal metabolic function. Including a mix of whole grains, lean proteins, healthy fats, fruits, and vegetables in your diet supports overall metabolic health.

3.2 Physical Activity and Exercise

3.2.1 Benefits of Regular Exercise

Physical activity and exercise are integral to metabolic health. Regular exercise offers numerous benefits, including improved insulin sensitivity, increased muscle mass, enhanced cardiovascular health, and weight management.

Exercise helps muscles become more sensitive to insulin, allowing them to use glucose more effectively for energy. This reduces the risk of insulin resistance and type 2 diabetes. Additionally, exercise increases the basal metabolic rate, leading to higher energy expenditure even at rest.

3.2.2 Types of Exercise for Metabolic Health

- **Aerobic Exercise**: Activities like jogging, cycling, and swimming increase cardiovascular fitness and enhance calorie burning. Aerobic exercise helps improve insulin sensitivity and supports weight management.

- **Resistance Training**: Lifting weights or using resistance bands builds muscle mass, which in turn increases the body's resting metabolic rate. More muscle tissue requires more energy to maintain, leading to higher calorie expenditure.

- **High-Intensity Interval Training (HIIT)**: HIIT involves short bursts of intense exercise followed by brief periods of rest. It's effective for burning calories, improving cardiovascular fitness, and promoting metabolic adaptations.

- **Flexibility and Balance Activities**: Practices like yoga and Pilates improve flexibility, balance, and overall well-being. While they may not have the same direct impact on metabolism as aerobic or resistance training, they contribute to an active lifestyle.

Diet, nutrition, and physical activity are fundamental factors influencing metabolic health. A balanced diet rich in macronutrients and micronutrients, along with avoiding excessive sugar and processed foods, is essential for maintaining metabolic balance. Regular exercise, encompassing a mix of aerobic, resistance, and flexibility activities, contributes significantly to improved metabolic function, weight management, and overall well-being.

3.3 Sleep and Stress

3.3.1 Sleep's Role in Metabolism

Sleep is a fundamental aspect of overall health and plays a significant role in metabolic processes. Adequate and quality sleep is crucial for maintaining metabolic balance, regulating hormones, and supporting optimal energy utilization.

During sleep, the body undergoes critical restorative processes, including the repair and growth of tissues. Sleep deprivation or poor sleep quality can disrupt hormonal balance, leading to changes in appetite-regulating hormones like leptin and ghrelin. This disruption often results in increased appetite and cravings for high-calorie, unhealthy foods.

Moreover, sleep deprivation can affect insulin sensitivity, leading to higher blood sugar levels and an increased risk of insulin resistance and type 2 diabetes. Chronic sleep deficiency has also been linked to weight gain, obesity, and a higher risk of cardiovascular diseases.

3.3.2 Managing Stress for Better Metabolic Health

Stress is an inherent part of life, but chronic stress can have a profound impact on metabolic health. When the body experiences stress, it releases hormones such as cortisol and adrenaline as part of the "fight or flight" response. In the short term, this response can be beneficial for survival. However, chronic stress can lead to sustained high levels of cortisol, disrupting metabolic processes.

Elevated cortisol levels can lead to increased appetite, particularly for high-calorie and sugary foods. This can contribute to weight gain and metabolic dysfunction. Chronic stress is also associated with increased inflammation, insulin resistance, and a higher risk of developing metabolic syndrome, a cluster of conditions that increase the risk of heart disease, stroke, and type 2 diabetes.

Managing stress through various techniques is essential for maintaining metabolic health:

- **Mindfulness and Meditation**: Practices that promote mindfulness and meditation can help reduce stress and improve emotional well-being. These techniques encourage relaxation and can positively impact cortisol levels.

- **Physical Activity**: Regular exercise not only has direct metabolic benefits but also acts as a stress-relieving activity. Engaging in physical activity releases endorphins, which are natural mood lifters.

- **Healthy Lifestyle Habits**: Adopting a balanced diet, getting enough sleep, and staying hydrated contribute to stress management and overall metabolic health.

- **Social Support**: Connecting with friends, family, or support groups can provide emotional support and help alleviate stress.

- **Time Management**: Efficiently managing time and prioritizing tasks can reduce feelings of being overwhelmed and stressed.

recognizing the role of sleep and stress in metabolic health is crucial for maintaining overall well-being. Prioritizing sufficient and restorative sleep, while effectively managing stress through various strategies, contributes to balanced hormonal regulation, improved appetite control, and better metabolic function.

CHAPTER 4

Assessing Your Metabolic Health

4.1 Measuring Body Composition

Assessing body composition is a valuable tool for understanding your metabolic health. Body composition refers to the proportions of different components in your body, such as lean muscle mass, body fat, bone, and water. Understanding these proportions helps you gain insights into your overall health and potential metabolic risk factors.

4.1.1 Body Mass Index (BMI) and its Limitations

Body Mass Index (BMI) is a common method used to assess body composition based on weight and height. While it provides a quick estimation of whether an individual is underweight, normal weight, overweight, or obese, BMI has limitations. It doesn't differentiate between muscle and fat, which can lead to inaccuracies, especially for individuals with high muscle mass. For instance, athletes or individuals who are muscular may have a higher BMI despite having low body fat.

Another limitation is that BMI doesn't consider the distribution of fat within the body. Central or visceral fat, which accumulates around the abdomen, is associated with a higher risk of metabolic disorders, such as type 2 diabetes and cardiovascular diseases. However, BMI doesn't take into account this important aspect of fat distribution.

4.1.2 Importance of Muscle Mass and Fat Percentage

Measuring muscle mass and body fat percentage provides a more comprehensive understanding of metabolic health. Muscle is metabolically active tissue that burns more calories at rest compared to fat. A higher muscle mass can enhance insulin sensitivity, improve metabolism, and support overall metabolic function.

Body fat percentage indicates the proportion of your body that is composed of fat. While some body fat is essential for energy storage and hormonal regulation, excess body fat, especially visceral fat, is associated with metabolic disturbances. Monitoring changes in body fat percentage over time can help track progress towards a healthier body composition.

Methods to measure muscle mass and body fat percentage include:

- **Dual-Energy X-ray Absorptiometry (DEXA)**: DEXA scans provide accurate measurements of bone density, lean mass, and body fat percentage.

- **Bioelectrical Impedance Analysis (BIA)**: BIA measures the resistance of body tissues to electrical currents, estimating body fat percentage and lean mass.

- **Skinfold Calipers**: Skinfold measurements at specific sites on the body can estimate body fat percentage.

- **Body Circumference Measurements**: Waist and hip measurements help assess fat distribution and the risk of central obesity.

Assessing body composition goes beyond just looking at weight and BMI. Understanding muscle mass, body fat percentage, and their distribution provides insights into your metabolic health and risk factors for various metabolic disorders. While BMI has its limitations, utilizing multiple methods to measure body composition can offer a more accurate picture of your overall health and guide your efforts to improve metabolic well-being.

4.2 Blood Tests and Biomarkers

Blood tests and biomarkers provide valuable insights into your metabolic health by assessing various physiological parameters. These tests help identify potential risks and provide a comprehensive view of your overall well-being.

4.2.1 Glucose Levels and Insulin Sensitivity

Monitoring blood glucose levels is crucial for assessing metabolic health. Elevated fasting blood glucose or impaired glucose tolerance may indicate insulin resistance, a condition where cells do not respond effectively to insulin's actions. This can lead to higher blood sugar levels and an increased risk of type 2 diabetes.

Additionally, measuring insulin sensitivity helps evaluate how well your body responds to insulin. Higher insulin sensitivity is associated with better metabolic health and a reduced risk of metabolic disorders. Various tests, such as the fasting insulin test or the homeostatic model assessment for insulin resistance (HOMA-IR), provide insights into your insulin sensitivity.

4.2.2 Lipid Profile and Heart Health

A lipid profile assesses the levels of different types of lipids (fats) in your blood. This profile includes measurements of total cholesterol, LDL cholesterol (often referred to as "bad" cholesterol), HDL cholesterol ("good" cholesterol), and triglycerides.

Elevated LDL cholesterol and triglyceride levels, along with low HDL cholesterol levels, can increase the risk of heart disease. LDL cholesterol can accumulate in arteries, leading to plaque formation and narrowing of blood vessels, a condition known as atherosclerosis. Monitoring your lipid profile helps identify potential cardiovascular risks and provides insight into your metabolic health.

4.2.3 Inflammation Markers and Metabolic Health

Chronic low-grade inflammation is closely linked to metabolic disorders. Inflammation markers such as C-reactive protein (CRP) and interleukin-6 (IL-6) can indicate the presence of inflammation in the body. Elevated levels of these markers are associated with an increased risk of insulin resistance, type 2 diabetes, and cardiovascular diseases.

Inflammation can also disrupt hormonal balance and contribute to the development of metabolic syndrome. Assessing inflammation markers can provide insights into your metabolic health status and guide interventions to reduce inflammation through lifestyle changes.

Blood tests and biomarkers are valuable tools for assessing metabolic health. Monitoring glucose levels, insulin sensitivity, lipid profile, and inflammation markers helps identify potential risks and provides a comprehensive view of your metabolic well-being. Regular screening and collaboration with healthcare professionals can help you understand your metabolic status and make informed decisions to support optimal health.

CHAPTER 5

Building Healthy Metabolic Habits

5.1 Designing a Balanced Diet

Creating a balanced diet is a foundational step towards improving metabolic health. A well-designed diet provides the necessary nutrients for optimal metabolic function, energy production, and overall well-being.

5.1.1 Portion Control and Mindful Eating

Portion control is a key aspect of maintaining a balanced diet. Overeating can lead to excess calorie intake, weight gain, and metabolic disturbances. Mindful eating, which involves paying attention to hunger cues and eating with intention, supports portion control and fosters a healthier relationship with food.

Practical tips for portion control and mindful eating include:

- **Eating slowly**: Savor each bite and give your body time to signal when you're full.

- **Using smaller plates and bowls**: This can help visually control portion sizes.

- **Listening to your body**: Eat when you're hungry and stop when you're satisfied, rather than finishing everything on your plate.

5.1.2 Incorporating Whole Foods

Whole foods are nutrient-dense and provide essential vitamins, minerals, fiber, and antioxidants. Incorporating whole foods into your diet supports metabolic health by providing sustained energy, supporting digestion, and reducing the risk of chronic diseases.

Focus on:

- **Fruits and Vegetables**: These are rich in vitamins, minerals, and fiber. They can help regulate blood sugar levels, support digestion, and provide antioxidants that combat oxidative stress.

- **Lean Proteins**: Incorporate sources like lean meats, poultry, fish, eggs, legumes, and tofu. Protein supports muscle maintenance, satiety, and energy balance.

- **Complex Carbohydrates**: Choose whole grains like quinoa, brown rice, and whole wheat. These carbohydrates provide steady energy and are higher in fiber, promoting digestive health.

- **Healthy Fats**: Opt for sources like avocados, nuts, seeds, and olive oil. Healthy fats support cell structure, hormone production, and overall metabolic function.

- **Hydration**: Staying hydrated with water and herbal teas is crucial for metabolic processes and overall health.

Designing a balanced diet involves portion control, mindful eating, and incorporating a variety of nutrient-dense whole foods. These practices promote metabolic health by providing essential nutrients, supporting steady energy levels, and aiding digestion. By making informed food choices and adopting mindful eating habits, you can build a foundation for better metabolic well-being.

5.2 Physical Activity and Exercise

Physical activity and exercise play a crucial role in improving metabolic health. Engaging in regular physical activity helps boost metabolism, enhance insulin sensitivity, and support overall well-being.

5.2.1 Setting Realistic Goals

Setting realistic goals is essential for establishing a sustainable exercise routine. Unrealistic expectations can lead to burnout and discouragement. When setting exercise goals, consider your current fitness level, time availability, and preferences.

Tips for setting realistic exercise goals:

- **Start Small**: Begin with manageable goals that align with your current fitness level. Gradually increase the intensity, duration, or frequency as you progress.

- **Be Specific**: Define clear and achievable goals. For example, aim to walk 30 minutes a day, three times a week, or to complete a certain number of steps each day.

- **Consider Your Lifestyle**: Choose activities that fit into your daily routine and are sustainable over the long term.

- **Track Your Progress**: Keep a record of your workouts and milestones. Tracking your progress can be motivating and help you stay on track.

5.2.2 Finding Activities You Enjoy

Finding enjoyable activities increases the likelihood that you'll stick to an exercise routine. Exercise doesn't have to mean spending hours in the gym; there are various options that can suit your interests and preferences.

Ideas for enjoyable physical activities:

- **Walking or Hiking**: A simple and effective way to stay active while enjoying nature.

- **Dancing**: Whether it's joining a dance class or dancing at home, it's a fun way to get moving.

- **Cycling**: Exploring your surroundings on a bike can be both enjoyable and beneficial for your metabolism.

- **Group Classes**: Joining fitness classes like yoga, Pilates, or aerobics can provide structure and social interaction.

- **Sports**: Engaging in sports like tennis, basketball, or swimming can make exercise feel like play.

- **Home Workouts**: Online workout videos and apps offer a wide range of options for exercising at home.

- **Gardening**: Gardening involves physical activity and can be a relaxing way to stay active.

Choosing activities, you enjoy increases your chances of staying consistent and making exercise a regular part of your lifestyle. Remember that variety is key; mixing different activities can prevent boredom and provide a balanced approach to physical fitness.

Physical activity and exercise are essential for improving metabolic health. Setting realistic goals and finding enjoyable activities help you establish a sustainable exercise routine. By making exercise a positive and fulfilling experience, you can support your metabolic well-being and overall health.

5.3 Prioritizing Sleep and Stress Management

5.3.1 Sleep Hygiene Tips

Sleep hygiene refers to practices that promote restful and rejuvenating sleep. Establishing healthy sleep habits can improve sleep quality and enhance metabolic health.

Effective sleep hygiene practices include:

- **Consistent Sleep Schedule**: Go to bed and wake up at the same time each day, even on weekends. This helps regulate your body's internal clock.

- **Create a Sleep-Conducive Environment**: Ensure your sleep environment is comfortable, dark, and quiet. Consider using blackout curtains and removing electronic devices that emit light.

- **Limit Screen Time Before Bed**: The blue light emitted by screens can interfere with your body's production of melatonin, a hormone that regulates sleep.

- **Mindful Eating Before Bed**: Avoid heavy meals close to bedtime. Opt for light, easily digestible snacks if necessary.

- **Regular Physical Activity**: Regular exercise can improve sleep quality, but avoid vigorous activity close to bedtime.

- **Relaxation Techniques**: Engage in relaxing activities before bed, such as reading, gentle yoga, or meditation, to prepare your mind for sleep.

- **Limit Caffeine and Alcohol**:
These substances can disrupt sleep
patterns. Avoid consuming them
close to bedtime.

- **Manage Stress**: High stress levels
can interfere with sleep. Engage in
stress-reducing activities
throughout the day.

5.3.2 Relaxation Techniques for Stress

Chronic stress can have detrimental
effects on metabolic health. Engaging
in relaxation techniques can help
manage stress levels and promote
overall well-being.

Effective relaxation techniques
include:

- **Deep Breathing**: Practice deep,
slow breathing to activate the

body's relaxation response and reduce stress.

- **Progressive Muscle Relaxation**: This involves tensing and then relaxing different muscle groups to release physical tension.

- **Mindfulness Meditation**: Focus your attention on the present moment, reducing rumination and promoting relaxation.

- **Yoga**: Gentle yoga poses and stretches can help alleviate physical tension and calm the mind.

- **Guided Imagery**: Visualize calming and peaceful scenes to shift your focus away from stressors.

- **Aromatherapy**: Certain scents, like lavender or chamomile, are believed to have relaxing effects.

- **Spending Time in Nature**: Being outdoors and connecting with nature can have a calming effect on the mind.

incorporating these relaxation techniques into your routine, you can effectively manage stress and support your metabolic health.

Prioritizing sleep and managing stress are vital for promoting metabolic health. Adopting sleep hygiene practices and engaging in relaxation techniques can improve sleep quality and reduce stress levels. These habits contribute to hormonal balance, appetite regulation, and overall well-being, enhancing your metabolic health journey.

CHAPTER 6

Meal Planning for Metabolic Health

6.1 The Importance of Meal Timing

Meal timing, or when you eat throughout the day, plays a significant role in supporting metabolic health. The timing of meals can influence various physiological processes, including insulin sensitivity, blood sugar regulation, and energy metabolism.

6.1.1 Circadian Rhythms and Meal Timing

The body operates on a natural 24-hour rhythm known as the circadian rhythm. This rhythm influences various biological processes, including hormone production, metabolism, and sleep-wake cycles. Meal timing that aligns with your circadian rhythm can have positive effects on metabolic health.

Key points about circadian rhythms and meal timing:

- **Breakfast**: Eating a balanced breakfast in the morning helps kickstart your metabolism and provides energy for the day ahead. It can also regulate hunger and prevent overeating later in the day.

- **Lunch**: Consuming a nutritious lunch helps maintain stable blood sugar levels and provides sustained energy throughout the afternoon.

- **Dinner**: Eating a lighter dinner earlier in the evening gives your body time to digest before sleep. Late-night eating can disrupt sleep and may lead to less effective digestion.

6.1.2 Impact of Meal Timing on Insulin Sensitivity

The body's response to insulin, a hormone that regulates blood sugar levels, can be influenced by meal timing. Consuming carbohydrates earlier in the day when insulin sensitivity tends to be higher can improve blood sugar control.

Key points about meal timing and insulin sensitivity:

- **Carbohydrates**: Distributing carbohydrate-rich meals earlier in the day can reduce post-meal blood sugar spikes and improve insulin sensitivity.

- **Avoiding Large Evening Meals**: Consuming large amounts of carbohydrates at night may lead to higher blood sugar levels and reduced insulin sensitivity the following morning.

6.1.3 The Role of Intermittent Fasting

Intermittent fasting is an eating pattern that alternates between periods of eating and fasting. It has gained attention for its potential benefits on metabolic health. Some forms of intermittent fasting, such as time-restricted feeding, focus on restricting the eating window to a specific time frame each day.

Key points about intermittent fasting and meal timing:

- **Insulin Sensitivity**: Intermittent fasting may improve insulin sensitivity and support blood sugar regulation.

- **Circadian Alignment**: Time-restricted feeding aligns eating with the body's natural circadian rhythm, potentially enhancing metabolic processes.

- **Individual Considerations**: Intermittent fasting approaches should be tailored to individual preferences and needs. Consulting a healthcare professional is recommended before making significant changes to your eating patterns.

Meal timing is an important aspect of promoting metabolic health. Aligning meals with circadian rhythms and focusing on distributing carbohydrates earlier in the day can positively impact blood sugar regulation and insulin sensitivity. Additionally, considering approaches like intermittent fasting under the guidance of a healthcare professional may offer benefits for metabolic well-being.

6.2 Building Balanced Meals

Creating balanced meals is essential for optimizing metabolic health. Well-rounded meals that include a mix of macronutrients provide sustained energy, support hormone regulation, and promote overall well-being.

6.2.1 Protein, Carbohydrates, and Fats

Balanced meals should incorporate the three main macronutrients: protein, carbohydrates, and fats. Each macronutrient serves a specific role in metabolism and overall health.

6.2.1.1 Protein

Protein is crucial for muscle repair, immune function, and hormone production. Including adequate protein in your meals can support satiety, prevent muscle loss, and enhance metabolic function.

Sources of protein include:

- Lean meats (chicken, turkey, lean cuts of beef or pork)

- Fish and seafood

- Eggs

- Dairy products (Greek yogurt, cottage cheese)

- Plant-based sources (beans, lentils, tofu, tempeh, quinoa)

6.2.1.2 Carbohydrates

Carbohydrates are the body's primary source of energy. Choose complex carbohydrates, which are rich in fiber and release energy gradually, to avoid blood sugar spikes and crashes.

Sources of complex carbohydrates include:

- Whole grains (brown rice, quinoa, whole wheat)

- Fruits (berries, apples, citrus fruits)

- Vegetables (leafy greens, broccoli, sweet potatoes)

- Legumes (beans, lentils, chickpeas)

6.2.1.3 Fats

Healthy fats are essential for cell structure, hormone production, and energy storage. Focus on unsaturated fats, which have heart-protective benefits.

Sources of healthy fats include:

- Avocado

- Nuts and seeds (almonds, walnuts, chia seeds)

- Olive oil

- Fatty fish (salmon, mackerel, sardines)

6.2.2 Planning Snacks for Sustained Energy

Balanced snacks can provide sustained energy between meals and prevent overeating during main meals. Choose snacks that combine protein, healthy fats, and fiber-rich carbohydrates for a well-rounded option.

Ideas for balanced snacks:

- Greek yogurt with berries and a sprinkle of nuts/seeds

- Apple slices with almond butter

- Carrot sticks with hummus

- Whole grain crackers with cheese

- Trail mix with dried fruits and nuts/seeds

- Cottage cheese with sliced peaches

Building meals that include a mix of protein, carbohydrates, and healthy fats, and incorporating balanced snacks, you can support steady energy levels, enhance metabolic function, and maintain overall well-being.

Building balanced meals that include protein, carbohydrates, and healthy fats is crucial for metabolic health. These macronutrients provide energy, support hormone regulation, and promote optimal physiological function. Additionally, planning balanced snacks can help sustain energy levels and prevent overeating.

6.3 Hydration and Its Role in Metabolism

Hydration is a fundamental aspect of metabolic health that often goes overlooked. Staying adequately hydrated supports various physiological processes, including digestion, nutrient transport, and energy metabolism.

6.3.1 Importance of Hydration

Proper hydration is essential for metabolic processes to function optimally. Water is involved in breaking down and absorbing nutrients from the foods you eat. It's also crucial for transporting nutrients and oxygen to cells and removing waste products from the body.

Key points about hydration and its importance:

- **Digestion and Nutrient Absorption**: Adequate hydration supports the breakdown of food and absorption of nutrients in the digestive system.

- **Thermoregulation**: Water helps regulate body temperature during metabolic processes, preventing overheating.

- **Energy Production**: Hydration supports cellular processes involved in energy production and metabolism.

6.3.2 Hydration and Weight Management

Hydration can also play a role in weight management and appetite regulation. Drinking water before meals can contribute to a feeling of fullness, potentially reducing overeating.

Key points about hydration and weight management:

- **Satiety**: Drinking water before meals can help control portion sizes and prevent overconsumption of calories.

- **Thirst vs. Hunger**: Sometimes, thirst can be mistaken for hunger.

Staying hydrated may help differentiate between the two sensations.

6.3.3 Tips for Staying Hydrated

Ensuring you're properly hydrated throughout the day is crucial for metabolic health. Here are some hydration tips:

- **Drink Water Regularly**: Aim to drink water consistently throughout the day, rather than waiting until you're thirsty.

- **Monitor Urine Color**: The color of your urine can be an indicator of hydration. Clear to pale yellow urine usually indicates proper hydration.

- **Incorporate Hydrating Foods**: Foods with high water content, such as fruits and vegetables, contribute to your overall hydration.

- **Drink Before, During, and After Exercise**: Hydrate before, during, and after physical activity to replace fluids lost through sweating.

- **Limit Sugary and Caffeinated Beverages**: While beverages like soda and certain types of coffee can contribute to hydration, they often come with added sugars and caffeine. Plain water is the best choice for hydration.

Hydration is a vital component of metabolic health. Proper hydration supports digestion, nutrient absorption, energy production, and weight management. Staying hydrated by drinking water regularly and

incorporating hydrating foods helps
maintain optimal metabolic function
and overall well-being.

CHAPTER 7

Long-Term Strategies for Sustainable Metabolic Health

7.1 Maintaining Consistency Over Time

Achieving and maintaining metabolic health requires consistency and a long-term approach. Sustainable habits and routines contribute to lasting improvements in metabolic function and overall well-being.

7.1.1 The Power of Consistency

Consistency is key to creating lasting changes in your metabolic health. Rather than relying on short-term solutions, developing consistent habits supports metabolic balance over time.

Key points about maintaining consistency:

- **Gradual Changes**: Slowly incorporating new habits allows you to adapt and make sustainable adjustments to your lifestyle.

- **Small Steps**: Focus on making manageable changes that are more likely to become permanent habits.

- **Lifestyle Integration**: Integrate healthy habits seamlessly into your daily routine, making them a natural part of your lifestyle.

7.1.2 Building a Routine

Establishing a routine helps reinforce healthy habits and provides structure for your daily activities. Routines can reduce decision fatigue and make it easier to prioritize actions that support your metabolic health.

Key points about building a routine:

- **Meal Times**: Try to eat meals at consistent times to regulate hunger and maintain stable blood sugar levels.

- **Scheduled Workouts**: Plan regular exercise sessions and prioritize physical activity, even on busy days.

- **Sleep Schedule**: Maintain a consistent sleep schedule to

support your body's natural
circadian rhythm.

7.1.3 Monitoring Progress

Regularly monitoring your progress
and making adjustments as needed is
essential for sustainable metabolic
health. Tracking your habits and
results helps you stay accountable and
make informed decisions.

Key points about monitoring
progress:

- **Journaling**: Keep a food and
  exercise journal to track your
  habits, emotions, and progress.

- **Periodic Assessments**: Schedule
  regular check-ins with your
  healthcare provider to assess your
  metabolic health and adjust your
  strategies as needed.

- **Celebrate Achievements**:
Acknowledge your successes and
milestones along the way to stay
motivated.

7.1.4 Staying Motivated

Maintaining motivation is a crucial
aspect of sustaining healthy habits for
metabolic health. Finding intrinsic
sources of motivation and setting
meaningful goals can help you stay on
track.

Key points about staying motivated:

- **Set Meaningful Goals**: Define
clear goals that are meaningful to
you, whether they involve
improved energy levels, weight
loss, or overall well-being.

- **Celebrate Non-Scale Victories**:
Focus on the positive changes you

experience beyond just the numbers on the scale.

- **Mindset Shift**: Shift your perspective from short-term results to the long-term benefits of consistent healthy habits.

Maintaining consistency over time is a foundational strategy for sustainable metabolic health. Gradual changes, building routines, monitoring progress, and staying motivated contribute to lasting improvements in your metabolic function and overall well-being. By prioritizing long-term habits, you can support your metabolic health journey for years to come.

7.2 Overcoming Challenges and Setbacks

On the journey to metabolic health, challenges and setbacks are inevitable. Learning how to overcome these obstacles and navigate setbacks is crucial for maintaining progress and staying committed to your goals.

7.2.1 Understanding Setbacks

Setbacks are temporary deviations from your desired path. They can include missed workouts, unhealthy food choices, or periods of low motivation. It's important to recognize that setbacks are a natural part of any journey and don't define your overall progress.

Key points about setbacks:

- **Normalizing Setbacks**:
  Understand that everyone faces
  challenges and setbacks on their
  health journey.

- **Opportunities for Learning**:
  Setbacks provide opportunities to
  learn and grow. Reflect on what
  led to the setback and how you can
  prevent it in the future.

- **Avoiding Self-Criticism**: Avoid
  negative self-talk or self-blame.
  Instead, practice self-compassion
  and focus on getting back on track.

7.2.2 Strategies for Overcoming Challenges

Successfully overcoming challenges
involves developing strategies to
navigate difficult situations and
setbacks. These strategies can help
you stay focused and motivated in the
face of adversity.

Key strategies for overcoming challenges:

- **Problem-Solving**: Analyze the challenge and brainstorm practical solutions. For example, if time constraints are hindering your workouts, consider shorter, high-intensity sessions.

- **Seeking Support**: Reach out to friends, family, or a support group for encouragement and accountability.

- **Setting Realistic Expectations**: Adjust your expectations to align with your current circumstances. It's okay to take smaller steps if that's what you can manage at the moment.

- **Reframing Negative Thoughts**: Transform negative thoughts into positive or constructive ones. For

instance, replace "I failed" with
"I'm learning and growing."

7.2.3 Cultivating Resilience

Resilience is the ability to bounce back from challenges and setbacks. Cultivating resilience enhances your capacity to cope with difficulties and continue working towards your metabolic health goals.

Key points about cultivating resilience:

- **Mindset Shift**: Embrace setbacks as opportunities for growth rather than as failures.

- **Focus on Progress**: Recognize the progress you've made, no matter how small, and use it as motivation to keep moving forward.

- **Practice Self-Care**: Engage in self-care activities that help you recharge and manage stress.

- **Stay Committed**: Remind yourself of your long-term goals and the importance of maintaining your health.

Overcoming challenges and setbacks is an integral part of the journey to metabolic health. Recognize setbacks as temporary deviations, develop strategies to navigate challenges, and cultivate resilience to stay committed to your goals. With the right mindset and practical approaches, you can overcome obstacles and continue making progress towards lasting metabolic well-being.

7.3 Seeking Professional Guidance

Seeking professional guidance is a pivotal step in your journey towards achieving and maintaining optimal metabolic health. While you can make significant progress by adopting healthy habits on your own, the expertise of qualified healthcare professionals can provide personalized insights, comprehensive assessments, and tailored recommendations that can make a substantial difference in your long-term success.

The Role of Healthcare Professionals:

1. **Registered Dietitians/Nutritionists:** These professionals specialize in nutrition and can create

personalized meal plans that align with your metabolic goals. They consider your dietary preferences, medical history, and lifestyle to develop an eating plan that supports your metabolic health. Dietitians also help you understand portion control, macronutrient distribution, and make informed food choices.

2. **Endocrinologists:** If you have concerns about hormonal imbalances affecting your metabolism, an endocrinologist is the right specialist to consult. They can diagnose and treat conditions like diabetes, thyroid disorders, and hormonal imbalances that impact your metabolic health.

3. **Fitness Trainers/Physical Therapists:** Collaborating with a fitness professional can be

immensely beneficial. They can design exercise routines tailored to your fitness level, age, and any underlying health conditions. Proper exercise helps improve insulin sensitivity, boost metabolism, and enhance cardiovascular health.

4. **Sleep Specialists:** If you struggle with sleep issues, consulting a sleep specialist can have a positive impact on your metabolic health. Sleep is closely linked to hormone regulation and metabolic function. Specialists can help address sleep disorders and provide guidance on improving sleep hygiene.

5. **Mental Health Professionals:** Managing stress and mental well-being is essential for metabolic health. Therapists and counselors can offer strategies for stress

management, relaxation techniques, and behavioral interventions that contribute to improved metabolic outcomes.

Benefits of Professional Guidance:

1. **Personalization:** Professionals tailor their guidance to your unique circumstances, considering factors like medical history, genetics, and lifestyle. This personalization increases the likelihood of sustained success.

2. **Accurate Assessment:** Healthcare professionals can conduct thorough assessments, including blood tests, body composition measurements, and metabolic rate evaluations. These assessments provide a clear understanding of your metabolic profile and any underlying issues.

3. **Evidence-Based Recommendations:** Professional guidance is rooted in evidence-based practices and the latest research. This ensures that the advice you receive is reliable and effective.

4. **Monitoring and Adjustments:** Professionals can monitor your progress over time and make necessary adjustments to your plan. This dynamic approach allows for continuous improvement and adaptation.

5. **Education:** Seeking guidance from professionals offers you the opportunity to learn about the science behind metabolic health. This knowledge empowers you to make informed decisions about your lifestyle choices.

How to Choose a Professional:

1. **Qualifications:** Ensure that the professional is qualified and certified in their respective field. Look for licenses, certifications, and relevant training.

2. **Experience:** Consider professionals with experience in dealing with metabolic health or related conditions. Experienced professionals are better equipped to provide accurate assessments and guidance.

3. **Compatibility:** A strong patient-professional relationship is crucial. Choose someone you feel comfortable talking to, as open communication is essential for effective guidance.

4. **Reviews and Recommendations:** Read reviews or seek

recommendations from trusted sources to gauge the experiences of others who have worked with the professional.

Seeking professional guidance for your metabolic health journey can be a game-changer. The expertise and personalized approach offered by healthcare professionals enhance your understanding of metabolic processes, optimize your health goals, and increase the likelihood of sustainable success. Remember that you are not alone on this journey – there are dedicated professionals ready to support you every step of the way.

7.4 Can Genetics Influence Metabolic Health?

Yes, genetics can play a significant role in influencing your metabolic health. While lifestyle factors such as diet, exercise, and sleep also contribute to your metabolic well-being, your genetic makeup can predispose you to certain metabolic characteristics and potential health outcomes. Understanding the interplay between genetics and metabolism can provide valuable insights into managing your health effectively.

Genetic Factors Impacting Metabolic Health:

1. **Metabolic Rate:** Your basal metabolic rate (BMR), which is the number of calories your body

needs at rest, can be influenced by genetics. Some individuals naturally have a higher BMR, making it easier for them to burn calories, while others have a lower BMR, making weight management more challenging.

2. **Fat Storage and Distribution:** Genetics can affect how your body stores and distributes fat. Some people may have a genetic tendency to store fat around the abdomen (central obesity), which is associated with a higher risk of metabolic disorders like type 2 diabetes and cardiovascular disease.

3. **Insulin Sensitivity:** Genetic factors can influence how sensitive your cells are to insulin, a hormone that regulates blood sugar levels. Reduced insulin sensitivity can

lead to insulin resistance and an increased risk of diabetes.

4. **Cholesterol Levels:** Your genes can impact your cholesterol levels, including LDL ("bad") cholesterol and HDL ("good") cholesterol. High LDL cholesterol and low HDL cholesterol levels are risk factors for heart disease.

5. **Blood Pressure:** Genetic variations can contribute to your susceptibility to high blood pressure (hypertension), a condition that is closely linked to metabolic health and cardiovascular risk.

6. **Metabolism of Nutrients:** Genetic variations can affect how your body processes and metabolizes nutrients, such as carbohydrates and fats. This can influence your

risk of weight gain, diabetes, and other metabolic disorders.

Gene-Environment Interaction:

It's important to note that genetics do not operate in isolation. Your genes interact with your environment, including your lifestyle choices, to determine your overall metabolic health. Even if you have genetic predispositions that might increase your risk of certain conditions, adopting a healthy lifestyle can help mitigate these risks.

Taking Action:

Understanding the role of genetics in metabolic health can empower you to make informed choices. Here's how:

1. **Personalized Approach:** Knowing your genetic predispositions can guide you in

tailoring your diet, exercise routine, and health management strategies to align with your unique needs.

2. **Early Intervention:** If you're aware of genetic factors that increase your risk of certain conditions, you can take proactive steps to prevent or manage them. Regular health screenings and check-ups are crucial.

3. **Focus on Lifestyle:** While genetics play a role, lifestyle factors like diet, exercise, sleep, and stress management have a substantial impact on your metabolic health. These factors are within your control and can help counteract genetic influences.

4. **Professional Guidance:** Genetic testing services and healthcare

professionals can offer insights into your genetic predispositions and provide guidance on how to optimize your health based on this information.

Genetics can indeed influence metabolic health by impacting factors such as metabolism, fat distribution, insulin sensitivity, and more. While genetics play a role, lifestyle choices remain a key determinant of overall metabolic well-being. By understanding your genetic predispositions and making informed lifestyle decisions, you can effectively manage and optimize your metabolic health.

www.ingramcontent.com/pod-product-compliance
Lightning Source LLC
Chambersburg PA
CBHW070836260726

48660CB00005B/2053